I0439461

Do-it-Yourself Homemade Skincare

Recipes for Masks, Scrubs, Soaps and Aromatherapy

Table of Contents

Disclaimer

All rights Reserved. No part of this publication or the information in it may be quoted from or reproduced in any form by means such as printing, scanning, photocopying or otherwise without prior written permission of the copyright holder.

Disclaimer and Terms of Use: Effort has been made to ensure that the information in this book is accurate and complete, however, the author and the publisher do not warrant the accuracy of the information, text and graphics contained within the book due to the rapidly changing nature of science, research, known and unknown facts and internet. This book is not meant to be taken as medical advice and consists only of the benefits that have been long known and shown by various research studies to be beneficial for human body. As always, before making any drastic changes to your regular diet or starting a special diet plan refer to your physician for advice. In case of allergic reaction, discontinue use of the product and consult your physician. The Author and the publisher do not hold any responsibility for errors, omissions or contrary interpretation of the subject matter herein. This book is presented solely for motivational and informational purposes only.

Copyright © 2014 by Sarah Reed

All Rights Reserved Worldwide

Welcome to "Do It Yourself Homemade Skin Care Recipes"

As the name of this book might suggest, it is all about creating natural, preservative and/or chemical free, and above all do it yourself homemade skincare products. At some point in our lives, we have all probably wondered what is in the food we eat and what is in the products we put on our faces and bodies on daily basis? If you were as curious as I was and you decided to do some research as to what all those fancy names under the ingredients portion of the lotion bottle were, you probably weren't happy about what you found out. I was shocked to find out that some of the products on my bathroom counter contained petroleum based dyes and flavors, flame retardants, emulsifiers, carcinogens such as 1,4 dioxane, polyethylene, just to name a few. Needless to say, my research was an eye opener on one hand and yet on the other hand it made me angry and upset at the manufacturers for fooling people into using their products when they can cause more harm than the benefits people hope for.

That anger became an inspiration for my experimentation with natural ingredients (often already found in our pantry) that could be used for natural and homemade skin or body-care products. I always heard from my mother that my aunt was using her own homemade concoctions as facemasks, scrubs, soaps, and even hair dyes. I also witnessed the result of her hard work of creating such DIY products in her well toned yet glowing skin and shiny hair. I always thought creating all those products on your own must be very cumbersome and time consuming and who has time for that? Well, I changed my priorities after finding out that I was putting on cancerous materials into my pores as moisturizers on daily basis, multiple times a day.

I wrote this book to share what I have found to be successful and effective homemade skin, body, and hair care products. In this book we are discussing the doom and gloom of your body and skin by sharing DIY secrets. This book is meant for all people who are interested in some natural treatment for their skin and hair. The basic ingredients for all recipes are simple to use and easy to make and I am sure you won't be surprised to find most of them already present in your kitchen pantry. Have you ever wondered when all these manufactured goods weren't available, what did people use to take care of their beauty and skincare needs? I am sure they weren't using petroleum based flame retardants to look pretty. Back in the day when life was simple, what existed in one's environment naturally was the answer to all the needs. Hence; we go back to nature for all we need to take care of our bodies.

This book comprises of four basic parts consisting of mask recipes, scrub recipes, homemade soaps and aromatherapy recipes. The recipes include masks for face, hand & feet, and hair. The skin care scrubs make the skin glow, soft and smooth. The hair mask recipes cover some effective ingredients leaving your hair much smoother, shinier and dandruff free. The homemade soaps are pure and organically made eliminating any harmful chemicals and also make a good use of essential oils. The aromatherapy recipes hide some astonishing results and give you a lot of freedom of using the essential oils you prefer to use.

But before getting started, if you are skeptical (as I myself was) as to why these homemade skincare products are beneficial for us and why choose these over some top brand name products which are usually endorsed by some celebrity (who is usually getting paid some big bucks for that endorsement) and testimonials we all often wonder about being real. I hope you will be convinced that natural is better than manufactured as your read on the benefits of natural homemade skin care products.

Benefits of Natural Homemade Skin Care Products

If you are a person who cares about your looks and you are a big fan of some branded masks that are readily available in a market, then you need to rethink. Many of the body, skin and hair care products that we use routinely, claim to be good for us but in fact they are harmful as they contain a lot of harmful and toxic chemical; lead to allergic reactions damaging hair and skin in long term. If we lean towards cheaper products, then quality is compromised again slowly hurting us in the long run. Unlike all the chemical filled stuff, natural and homemade organic products are a real deal for you. As organic and natural products are safer to use and contain no harmful chemicals and ingredients. Moreover, our bodies adhere to natural things and respond to natural ingredients more readily. All the natural ingredients are:

1. Chemical free
2. Contain no additive ingredients
3. Contain no toxic chemicals

4. More effective
5. No side effects
6. Zero damage (unless any allergies exits)
7. Natural means organic that means earth friendly
8. Inexpensive

After knowing the benefits of natural skin care products over the marketed ones, it's now time to get started with making some do-it-yourself, homemade, and natural facial, hand, feet, body scrubs, hair and face mask, soaps and aromatherapy products. You are sure to enjoy a little experimentation with the ingredients that are so readily available in your kitchen pantry and reap the benefits of natural products. Let's start the revitalization right in your own kitchen.

Homemade Soap Recipes

Soaps are in use on daily basis as cleaning products for hands, face, and body. Readymade soaps contain many harsh chemicals which in most cases leave our skin extremely dry and damaged. Many people among us feel the irritation from soap usage, often extremely dry skin is a result and people even get serious allergic reactions to the chemical content in commercially available soaps.

Homemade soap making is a great and easy solution to this problem. Homemade soap making is a great hobby as these soaps are natural with great aromas and benefits for the skin in long term. Moreover homemade soap are inexpensive and environment friendly. Homemade soaps are prepared from natural oils and ingredients that provide instant relief to sensitive skin.

If you are a first time soap maker or you are someone who has never thought of making soap at home before, I am providing you with the simplest method of homemade soap making known as Melt-and-Pour method. The recipes to follow will teach you basic steps of soap making with a lot of room for experimentation and creating your own personal favorite blends.

There are a variety of soap molds available in craft stores near you. Soap base and all other accessories are easily available in any craft store as well. So stock up or be creative and use anything you might find lying around in the house for a mold. You will be surprised at what you might find in your house, it doesn't have to be fancy. Some people often like to use small size rectangular cardboards lined with wax paper to make one big soap block and then just cut it into desired size bars. So you don't have to be fancy and it doesn't have to be expansive but you will really enjoy the hidden creativity inside you which is sure to come out with these simple homemade soap recipes.

Aromatherapy with Essential Oils

The recipes included in this portion are merely compiled to reduce stress and provide relaxation. Before introducing the recipes let's discuss the concept of aromatherapy. Aromatherapy uses some essential oils. These oils can be useful for health, beauty and physical hygiene. The inhalation of the aromatic oil can relax the brain and applying it to skin provides muscle relaxation, releases any tension and stress while reducing any pain.

Now that we have discussed all major sections of the book, let's begin the journey to natural beautification and relaxation!

Mask Recipes for Hair, Face, Hands, & Feet

Do not pay a lot for market bought masks; prepare some simple yet easy to make masks right at home by utilizing easily available every day ingredients.

Oatmeal and Onion Face Mask

This mask is good for acne prone skin. The oatmeal in itself is a very good cleanser and work great for exfoliation. Onions have some anti-inflammatory qualities which can be great for acne prone skin. Though, It does not promise a clear skin that is completely free of acne in the individuals with a hormonal imbalance, this mask can be used as a natural cleanser as it helps in cleansing your skin.

Ingredients

1/3 cup boiling water

1/2 cup plain oatmeal

1-2 white onion (chopped and refrigerated for at least 30 minutes prior to use, to avoid any onion induced tear production)

1 teaspoon of honey

Preparation

1. Place the oatmeal in boiling water and let it sit for 10 minutes in a bowl.

2. Add onions in the food processor and turn into a paste. Add honey to the onion paste.
3. Add the onion mixture into the oatmeal bowl. Mix well and then spread the mask on the face.
4. If the mask is not thick enough, more honey and oatmeal can be added till the desired consistency is created.

You can also refrigerate this mask if you plan to use it sometimes in future. However, onions might release some water resulting in more thin/watery consistency. So I do not recommend keeping this mask for too long. Also, the whole purpose of using natural ingredients is to utilize the benefits of fresh ingredients so personally I do not like to make and store such recipes for too long. The fresher it is the better. However, there is no harm per se if you were to refrigerate this recipe for a day or two. Just remember to warm it up slightly before applying to your face.

Homemade Clay Mask for All Skin Types

People with oily skin realize that it often does not look very appealing. Most women feel a great dissatisfaction when they lose the freshness of their makeup due to oily secretions and the foundation literally melts off of the face.

Clay masks are mostly used for oily skins and have a very soothing impact. This simple homemade clay mask works wonders. The results are long lasting and your skin will remain clean and clear for a long time. So get rid of your oily skin in summers and throughout the year. The ingredients of this mask are simple and need very less time to prepare.

Ingredients

2 tablespoons Green Clay (Bentonite Clay)

2-3 tablespoon of water

Directions & use:

1. Combine both of the listed ingredients until a homogenous paste is formed.
2. Gently layer it on your face or any other skin area of interest such as hands or top parts of feet.
3. Leave the mask on for 20-30 minutes or until the mask is dry.
4. Wash it off with warm water.

Modification for Normal & Dry Skin types:

In order to make this mask for normal skin type, replace water with milk.

If you have dry skin, then mix in jojoba oil instead of water or milk. The mask is great for any skin type with slight modifications.

P.S. Green clay might not be something we all have just lying around in the house. However, it is fairly easily available in most health stores or even online stores in powdered form.

Juice Mask for Oily Skin

This simple mask is prepared from juices of nutritious fruits like orange, lemon and strawberries. Lemons contain citric acid which cleanses the skin. Oranges provide nourishment and strawberries treat all the pimples and acne.

Ingredients

2 tablespoons lemon juice (freshly squeezed)

4 tablespoons orange juice (freshly squeezed from fruit)

1 strawberry

Directions and use:

1. Blend all the listed ingredients in a blender at slow speed for just a few seconds.
2. Once a thick concentrate is formed, gently massage the face with it. Leave the leftover paste on the skin for 15 minutes.
3. Wash your face with warm water. You will feel the difference in your skin right away as this mask will give your skin a glow.

Brightening Mask for Feet, Legs, Arms and Face for Darker Complexion

If you are tired of spending a lot of money on store bought creams which promise brighter glowing skin but such results are never realized; then try this homemade skin care treatment. You will begin to notice the results within one week of use. The recipe combines the turmeric powder with milk or yogurt. Turmeric is an Asian spice that can easily be bought from your local grocery stores. If for some reason you cannot find it in western grocery stores, Indian grocery stores are sure to have it on hand. The turmeric mask leaves the skin supple and soft.

Ingredients (for normal skin)

1 teaspoon turmeric

2 tablespoons of milk

2 tablespoon flour of your choice (rice flour, almond flour etc.) or ground oats.

1 tablespoon of Rose water (Optional, though it can be easily found in Indian grocery stores)

Directions & use:

1. Combine all the ingredients in a bowl. The paste should be creamy in texture.
2. Now gently message it on legs, arms or face.
3. Leave it on for 10 minutes and then wash the area with water.

Other Skin Types:

Dry Skin:

If you have dry skin, you can replace milk with olive, mustard, coconut or any other oil of preference.

Oily Skin:

For oily skin, replace milk with 1/4 cup of plain yogurt and apply. It can help with healing acne.

P.S. *This mask is not suited for fair skin, as the strong yellow color of turmeric will stain your skin. However, the stain is not long lasting and can be washed off easily. It is best suited to be used for darker complexion. However, the amount of turmeric can be reduced to reduce the yellowish tint possible from the use of turmeric.*

Banana Mask for Oily Skin

Banana mask is a soothing mask which can be prepared easily at home with some organic bananas. It is especially beneficial for oily skin.

Ingredients

1 fresh organic banana, ripe

4 teaspoons honey

Juice of one lemon

Directions & use:

1. Mash the banana with a fork in a bowl.
2. Mix in honey and lemon juice.
3. Combine all the ingredients well and then apply on face for 15 minutes then remove.
4. Wash your face with luke-warm water and pat dry.

Eggs, Yogurt & Coconut Oil Mask for Hair

This simple hair mask can give you amazingly soft and shiny hair with only once a weak use. We have all heard or seen how shiny new born babies' hair usually is. The chemicals found in placenta are similar to eggs. These chemicals have conditioning qualities and can work miracles on your hair. We might not have access to the placenta or we might be turned off by putting it on ourselves but egg is an easy alternative to placentas. Yogurt in this recipe is very soothing for the roots and scalp conditioning, which also assists with controlling the dandruff. On the other hand, egg in this mask acts as a natural conditioner resulting in soft and shinny hair just like a new born. Coconut oil has been used all over Asia for centuries for hair care and is considered very nutritive and conditioning for all hair types.

Ingredients

1 cup plain yogurt

2 eggs

2 to 3 Tablespoon Coconut oil

Directions & use:

1. Break both eggs into a bowl and whisk the yolks and egg whites completely.
2. Add the coconut oil to the egg and whisk together till mixed well.
3. Add the yogurt to the mixture and mix well.

4. Part your hair and apply the mixture concentrating on the scalp and roots.
5. Apply by parting the hair all over the scalp and massage in with your finger tips.
6. Leave the mask in the hair for at least 30 minutes.
7. Wash with shampoo and use conditioner. Presence of coconut oil egg warrants washing your hair 2 to 3 times in order to get all the ingredients out of your hair (Trust me it is worth the effort). Washing the hair with clarifying shampoo and luke-warm water works better.
8. After washing, wrap your hair in a towel and leave the towel turban on for 15 minutes before brushing.
9. Enjoy extremely soft and shiny hair.

P.S. This recipe can be modified by either eliminating the oil altogether or the coconut oil can be replaced by any other oil of choice such as mustard, olive, or even tea-tree oil. Use of tea-tree oil is very beneficial if head-lice are a problem.

Banana & Avocado Treatment for Dry Hair

If you are not a fan of chemical treatments for your hair then this homemade natural hair treatment is for you. The banana and avocado are not only great for skin but also for hair. Here is one recipe to treat damaged and dry hair.

Ingredients

1 banana, ripe

1 avocado, ripe

1 tablespoon of olive oil

A few drops of lavender oil

Directions & use:

1. Mash and combine all the ingredients in a blender until smooth.
2. Comb out and then apply this mask on hair and scalp.
3. Now put on a shower cap and let your hair sit covered under the shower cap for 25 minutes.
4. Rinse in the shower with shampoo and a conditioner.

Avocado, Olive Oil, & Egg Treatment for Dry Hair

Avocado is a natural moisturizer and conditioner for skin and hair as it contains many essential oils and vitamins. Avocado is full of many nutrients that can lead to healthy hair and this mask is especially beneficial for color-treated, dried, and damaged hair. This hair mask is just as beneficial for normal hair as well as it provides the hair with plenty of protein.

One more thing I always like to mention is that the key to the application of such masks and products to hair and skin isn't only the ingredients, though that is a major part however; the scalp and/or skin massage done during the application is just as critical. Good massage of the scalp increases the blood supply to the scalp and more blood means more oxygen, more nutrition which is equally important for healthy hair.

Ingredients

Pulp/meat of one ripe avocado (mashed)

1 Egg

2 Tablespoon Olive Oil (if you are not a fan, change it to any other oil you prefer e.g. Coconut oil)

Directions & use:

1. Mash the pulp of a ripe avocado in a bowl.
2. Beat one egg completely and add into the bowl of avocado pulp.

3. Add in the preferred oil and whisk all ingredients till a homogenous mixture is formed.
4. Apply to clean and dry hair while massaging the scalp well and leave it on for at least 1 hour.
5. Put on a shower cap over your hair to avoid staining any surroundings.
6. After the desired time, shampoo well and condition using your favorite conditioner.
7. Enjoy your soft and shiny hair.

Baking Soda Face Mask

This proven treatment has satisfied many people. If you are self-conscious about pimples on your skin and you do not have extra money to spend on expensive facemasks then try this simple treatment at home. This can be used as a spot treatment, concentrating on the areas with zits and pimples or the quantity can be increased to treat larger skin areas such as the entire face.

Ingredients

3 teaspoons Baking Soda

Water or lemon juice about 1 to 1 ½ teaspoons

How to Make and Use

1. Mix together the baking soda with water till a thick paste is formed.
2. Wash the face with warm water and pat dry with towel
3. Now apply this mask to acne prone areas and leave on for 20 minutes.
4. After 20 minutes, wash the area with warm water
5. Use this mask once a week in order to keep acne in check.

If there is an allergic reaction then do not use this treatment. Never use this home treatment too frequently as it can cause excess skin dryness. Avoid sun exposure after using this mask to avoid harmful effects to your skin.

Cucumber and Oats Facial Mask for Oily Skin

Cucumber is one of the best natural cleansers and it works perfectly with oats against aging. If you are suffering from acne and pimples then try this unique recipe. This mask helps fight acne, pimples, while exfoliating the skin at the same time. It helps with healing and nourishing the skin. This mask prevents the dull appearance of the skin by eliminating the dead skin from face. It is a perfectly nourishing body mask best suited for oily skin type.

Ingredients

1 cucumber, grated

1 tablespoons of oat

3 teaspoon juice of lemon

2 tablespoon of honey

How to Make and Use

1. Place the cucumber in a blender and blend until pureed.
2. Add in the oats, lemon juice and honey and blend till a homogenous mixture is formed.
3. Once the mask is ready, apply it to a washed face, legs or any skin area you want to treat.
4. Leave it on for 20 minutes then wash.
5. After the treatment, avoid sun exposure for few hours.

Egg White Mask for Skin and Hair

With just one simple ingredient, you can get the skin and hair of your dreams. That magic ingredient is the egg white. Egg whites are rich in an enzyme known as lysozyme which provides barrier against bacteria. It is also rich in protein and other essential nutrients which are essential for hair and skin health. Egg whites are also loaded with collagen which is important for skin renewal.

Ingredient

2 egg whites

How to Make and Use:

1. Whisk the egg whites until foamy .
2. Apply it to face, hand and legs, or hair. Apply the generous amount of egg white mixture on scalp and hairs.
3. Leave it on skin for 20 minutes. Leave it on hair for 30 minutes at least. You will feel the stiffness once the mask is dry.
4. Wash your skin or hair with luke-warm water and then tap dry with towel. This mask would leave your skin really soft. This mask also leaves the hair soft, conditioned, and shiny.

P.S. Another good use of egg white is using it as a first-aid for burns. Its high content of collagen help the burnt skin by providing it with desired nutrients needed to heal and renew the dead/burnt skin.Scrub Recipes

Scrub Recipes

Sugar Scrub

Too much sugar is not good for health but if used externally, it can work wonders on your skin. Try this sugar scrub for full body nourishment. This scrub will help exfoliate the skin and clean the pores while cleaning the skin in a gentle way

Ingredients

2 tablespoon brown sugar

1 tablespoons white sugar

2 tablespoons of Honey (Organic preferred)

2 tablespoons olive oil

How to Make and Use:

1. Combine all the listed ingredients and gently scrub on legs, arms and overall body.
2. Scrub more vigorously on areas prone to be really dry and dead skin such as elbows, knuckles etc.
3. Wash with soap and warm water and pat dry.
4. Apply your favorite moisturizer quickly in order to lock in the moisture and retain the softness.

Pumpkin Scrub

This pumpkin scrub is easy to make yet the results are quite amazing. Try the recipe yourself and feel the difference.

Ingredients

2 cups of brown sugar (packed)

2 tablespoons of vitamin E oil (or any other oil of choice e.g. coconut, olive)

2 teaspoons pumpkin pie spice

1 teaspoon of vanilla essence (organic)

½ teaspoon of nutmeg

1/3 cup of olive oil

How to make and use:

1. Combine all the listed ingredients to make the scrub. This recipe makes a larger batch of the scrub which can be stored in any glass jar with a lid for a long time.
2. In order to use this scrub, apply it to hands, arms, feet, and even face. However, scrubbing should be much gentle on face.
3. Gently message for 5 minute. Then leave for 5 additional minutes.
4. Then wash the area with warm water and pat dry.

5. This scrub not only makes your skin really soft and beautiful but it also smells delicious.

Brown Sugar, Honey & Lemon Scrub

This scrub is best to use after washing dishes. Here is the recipe for you.

Ingredients

½ cup brown sugar

2 tablespoon vitamin E oil

1 tablespoon honey

Juice of 1 to 2 lemons

Preparation:

1. Combine all the listed ingredients in a bowl.
2. Gently message on hands after washing the dishes.
3. It will leave your hands soft and smooth.
4. Use the scrub twice a day for best results.

Tip & Tricks:

Never throw away the lemon peel from the squeezed lemon. It is a great cleanser and moisturizer. Use the inside of the lemon peel (this side with juice pockets) and rub it on any area you would like to be soft and cleansed. Keep rubbing the peel all over the desired area, leave it on for a few minutes and wash with warm water. Your skin will be surprisingly soft after just one use.

Sea Salt Body Scrub

This scrub is an excellent detoxifying scrub to use. Ingredients are few but they can be easily accessed in your pantry.

Ingredients

½ cup of sea salt

1/4 cup of baby oil

How to Make and Use

1. Combine all the listed ingredients in a bowl.
2. Let the scrub sit for few hours so ingredient will mix better.
3. Mix well again right before use. Apply to your body in shower and message/scrub well for few minutes.
4. Rinse and get ready to experience a smooth skin

Coffee Scrub

Coffee is something we all drink daily but very few people know that it can be very beneficial for your skin if applied externally. Coffee has great anti-aging properties and if you want to get rid of cellulite then this simple recipe is for you. The ingredients are few and simple but lead to amazing results.

Ingredients

1/3 cup ground coffee beans

1 cup brown sugar

½ cup organic nut oil (Almond etc.)

Few drops of mint oil

Preparation:

1. Combine all the ingredients in a bowl.
2. Apply to body in the bathtub and message. Scrub vigorously on cellulite prone areas especially.
3. Wash with your favorite homemade soap/body wash, pat dry and apply good amount of moisturizer for prolonged softness.

P.S. Beware, coffee will stain white bathtubs so I suggest doing this when cleaning bathroom was already on the to-do list.

Olive Oil Scrub

Olive is not only good for health if used internally but it is also good for our skin, hair and face if used externally for cleansing or massage. You can use this scrub on feet. It is great for exfoliating and makes the skin baby soft and smooth. Olive oil is one of the best ingredients to use on skin as it reduces dryness in winter and helps in nourishing the skin while reducing wrinkles.

Ingredients

6 tbsp. extra virgin olive oil

1 tbsp. honey

1/3 cup sugar

Preparation

1. Combine all ingredients in a bowl and mix them using a spoon.
2. Apply to desired area and scrub vigorously.
3. Leave on the skin for 5 to 10 minutes.
4. Wash, rinse, & pat dry.

P.S. Olive oil is also a great cleanser as this is the only natural oil that does not clog pores. So if you are tired or lazy (like I am on many nights) reach for a cotton ball and olive oil to remove your make up. If you use any other kind of oil, you have to wash it off because it will clog your pores but that is not the case with olive oil.

Almond Orange Scrub

This is a perfect scrub with amazing benefits of almonds for skin. Almonds not only help with exfoliating the dead skin but they also revitalize the skin.

Ingredients

1 cup Almonds

3 teaspoons orange peel

1 Tablespoon Honey

¼ cup Milk

Preparation:

1. Combine all the ingredients and blend in a food processor.
2. Apply to the body in the shower and scrub/massage the skin.
3. Leave on the skin for at least 5 minutes.
4. Wash & Rinse.
5. Thoroughly moisturize after the shower.

Ginger and Coconut Oil Sugar Scrub

The combination of coconut oil and ginger helps in fighting the signs of wrinkles and dead skin.

Ingredient

½ cup coconut oil

2 tablespoons ginger (chopped)

½ cup almond oil

1/4 cup brown sugar

2 to 3 cups sea salt

4 drops essential oil of your choice

Preparation:

1. Take a pan and heat ginger in it for 10 minutes then add in coconut oil and turn off the heat.
2. Now pour it through a coffee filter and mix in the almond oil.
3. Stir in sugar, sea salt and mix well.
4. Add in essential oil once the temperature of the mixture is at the room temperature.
5. Apply to body and face once the temperature of the mixture is tolerable for the skin.
6. Wash & rinse after few minutes of scrubbing and pat dry.

Strawberry and Sugar Scrub

Strawberries are chock full of antioxidants which are important in removing impurities and free radicals from our body. Strawberries have a detoxification impact on our body so what better way to cleanse our skin than to use nature's very best cleansers like strawberries. This scrub makes your skin luscious and leaves it smelling delicious.

Ingredients

1 cup raw sugar (granulated or brown sugar)

1 cup olive oil

¾ cup strawberries

2 teaspoons honey

Preparation

1. Combine all ingredients in a blender and blend till a homogenous mixture is formed.
2. Apply on the face or all over the body in shower
3. . Message gently & leave it on for at least 5 minutes.
4. Rinse with warm water & pat dry.

Cinnamon & Nutmeg Scrub

This scrub recipe smells amazing and is perfect for cold winter days with its warm spice blend.

Ingredients

½ cup brown sugar

1/4 cup almond oil

2 teaspoons cinnamon

1 teaspoons ginger

2 teaspoons nutmeg

Preparation

1. Combine all ingredients in a bowl and mix well.
2. Apply to all over your body or face and massage vigorously for few minutes.
3. Rinse with warm water and pat dry.

Homemade Soap Recipes

These homemade soap recipes are sure to help find the hidden creativity inside you. These recipes follow the simplest method of soap making and your imagination can take you on a wild ride of creating healthy and aromatic DIY homemade soaps.

Goat Milk, Mint, & Green Tea Soap

Ingredients

2lb Goat milk Melt & Pour soap base

2 tablespoon honey

2 Tea bags of Green tea

¼ teaspoon mint fragrance (or essential oil if preferred)

Spray bottle with rubbing alcohol

Preferred mold

Yield: 8 bars (will depend on size of mold used)

Preparation:

1. Cut the 2lb goat milk melt and pour soap base into smaller chunks & put them in a microwave safe beaker/dish.

2. Follow the manufacturer's directions for melting in the microwave. I mostly melt the base in increments of 1 minute at a time initially. Run the microwave for 1 minute, stir the base and run for another 1 minute. When most of the base has been softened and has begun to melt, change the increments to be 30 seconds.
3. Melt the base for 30 second increments stir and continue to heat up in microwave until the entire base has been melted.
4. Open the tea bags and add the tea leaves to the melted base.
5. Add honey and the fragrance and mix all the ingredients well while mixing gently.
6. Pour the mixture into the molds. Spray alcohol on top of each mold in order to remove any air bubbles that might gather on top. Let it cool for at least 6 hours or until the soap base is completely solid again.
7. Remove from the molds and wrap each bar with your favorite tissues and twine. These make great presents as well.

Oatmeal, Honey, & Goat Milk Soap

This soap is bound to leave your skin silky smooth as the goat milk will moisturize your skin while it is being washed and the oats can have an exfoliating function as part of this combination.

Ingredients

2lb Goat milk Melt & Pour soap base

3 tablespoon honey

1 cup Ground Oats

¼ teaspoon Vanilla fragrance (or essential oil if preferred)

Spray bottle with rubbing alcohol

Preferred mold

Yield: 8 bars (will depend on size of mold used)

Preparation:

1. Cut the 2lb goat milk melt and pour soap base into smaller chunks & put them in a microwave safe beaker/dish.
2. Follow the manufacturer's directions for melting in the microwave. I mostly melt the base in increments of 1 minute at a time initially. Run the microwave for 1 minute, stir the base and run for another 1 minute. When most of the base has been softened and has begun to melt, change the increments to be 30 seconds.

3. Melt the base for 30 second increments, stir and continue to heat up in microwave until the entire base has been melted.
4. Add honey, ground oats and the fragrance in the melted base. Mix all the ingredients well but do so gently.
5. Pour the mixture into the molds. Spray alcohol on top of each mold in order to remove any air bubbles that might gather on top. Let it cool for at least 6 hours or until the soap base is completely solid again.
6. Remove from the molds and wrap each bar with your favorite tissues and twine.

Orange Poppy Seed Goat Milk Soap

Nothing can make you feel more fresh and invigorating than the scent of citrus fruits. This soap with orange zest does exactly that. The clean and sweet scent of orange along with the exfoliating qualities of poppy seeds in addition to moisturizing goat milk work in perfect harmony and will make your body scream for more.

Ingredients

2lb Goat milk Melt & Pour soap base

2 tablespoon Poppy seeds

Zest of 4 Oranges

2 teaspoons Orange fragrance/essential oil

Spray bottle with rubbing alcohol

Preferred mold

Yield: 8 bars (will depend on size of mold used)

Preparation

1. Cut the 2lb goat milk melt and pour soap base into smaller chunks & put them in a microwave safe beaker/dish.
2. Follow the manufacturer's directions for melting in the microwave. I mostly melt the base in increments of 1 minute at a time initially. Run the microwave for 1 minute, stir the base and

run for another 1 minute. When most of the base has been softened and has begun to melt, change the increments to be 30 seconds.

3. Melt the base for 30 second increments, stir and continue to heat up in microwave until the entire base has been melted.

4. Add Orange zest, poppy seeds and the fragrance in the melted base. Mix all the ingredients well but do so gently.

5. Pour the mixture into the molds. Spray alcohol on top of each mold in order to remove any air bubbles that might gather on top. Let it cool for at least 6 hours or until the soap base is completely solid again.

6. Remove from the molds and wrap each bar with your favorite tissues and twine.

Goat Milk & Lavender Soap

Lavender is most often used in herbal spa treatment because of the stress releasing qualities hidden associated with its fragrance. A nice warm bath with this goat milk and lavender soap is sure to send you off to a great night sleep.

Ingredients

2lb Goat milk Melt & Pour soap base

1 cup Lavender (Fresh is great but if you have it in dry form, it works just as great)

2 teaspoons Lavender fragrance/essential oil

Spray bottle with rubbing alcohol

Preferred mold

Yield: 8 bars (will depend on size of mold used)

Preparation

1. Cut the 2lb goat milk melt and pour soap base into smaller chunks & put them in a microwave safe beaker/dish.
2. Follow the manufacturer's directions for melting in the microwave. I mostly melt the base in increments of 1 minute at a time initially. Run the microwave for 1 minute, stir the base and run for another 1 minute. When most of the base has been softened and has begun to melt, change the increments to be 30 seconds.

3. Melt the base for 30 second increments, stir and continue to heat up in microwave until the entire base has been melted.
4. Add lavender and the fragrance in the melted base. Mix all the ingredients well but do so gently.
5. Pour the mixture into the molds. Spray alcohol on top of each mold in order to remove any air bubbles that might gather on top. Let it cool for at least 6 hours or until the soap base is completely solid again.
6. Remove from the molds and wrap each bar with your favorite tissues and twine.

Amaretto Coffee Bean Soap

Once again, this soap is a 2 in one combination. Goat milk is a great moisturizer and coffee beans exfoliate polishing away the dead skin cells. The almond fragrance is a good wake me up in addition to the aroma of coffee beans in this soap. This is a must have recipe you are sure to enjoy in your daily morning routine.

Ingredients

2lb Goat milk Melt & Pour soap base

1 ½ cup ground coffee beans

2 tablespoon whole coffee beans (optional- makes the soap more eye catching)

3 teaspoons Almond fragrance/essential oil

Spray bottle with rubbing alcohol

Preferred mold

Yield: 8 bars (will depend on size of mold used)

Preparation

1. Cut the 2lb goat milk melt and pour soap base into smaller chunks & put them in a microwave safe beaker/dish.
2. Follow the manufacturer's directions for melting in the microwave. I mostly melt the base in increments of 1 minute at a time initially. Run the microwave for 1 minute, stir the base and

run for another 1 minute. When most of the base has been softened and has begun to melt, change the increments to be 30 seconds.

3. Melt the base for 30 second increments, stir and continue to heat up in microwave until the entire base has been melted.

4. Add ground coffee, whole coffee beans and the fragrance in the melted base. Mix all the ingredients well but do so gently.

5. Pour the mixture into the molds. Spray alcohol on top of each mold in order to remove any air bubbles that might gather on top. Let it cool for at least 6 hours or until the soap base is completely solid again.

6. Remove from the molds and wrap each bar with your favorite tissues and twine.

Aromatherapy with Essential Oils Recipes

Let me introduce you to some very easy home based aromatherapy recipes to get you started on your journey to create your home-spa and be stress free.

For Relaxation

4 drops Lavender essential oil

4 drops Tangerine essential oil

4 drops Marjoram essential oil

2 drop Chamomile essential oil

Directions:

Combine all of the above oils and message on the desired areas to reduce stress. This particular combination provides relaxation to joints, muscles and relieves headache.

Bath Musk

1/3 cup aloe gel

1/4 cup honey

1/2 cup sea or rock salt

2 tablespoons of jojoba essential oil (optional)

5 drops lavender oil

Directions:

Specifically made to work during the bath time. All these ingredients can be added to a bath tub full of warm water. If you plant to relax and take a long bath, just add these ingredients to your bath and let your body soak in this magic potion. A perfect blend made for bath that provides soothing effect to overall body. It leaves your skin soft and smooth. You can also just use the blend to massage the body before getting in the warm bath.

Rosemary Mist

This Rosemary mist is used to relax and provide relaxing sensation to the brain. A perfect post shower mist, that is surprisingly easy to make.

Ingredients

5 ounces distilled water

1 tsp olive oil

6 drops rosemary essential oil

1 sprig fresh rosemary.

How to use

Shake well to mix and then spray on as desired.

(*To be sprayed on the skin and not cloths as the oils might stain the fabric*)

Cold and Flu Fighter

Ingredients

5 drops of Eucalyptus essential oil

5 drops Scotch pine essential oil

5 drops Lemon essential oil

Big pot of boiling water

How to make and use

Combine all the listed ingredients and then add them to a large bowl of steaming water. Now cover the head and pan with a towel falling over your head and the pot to seal in the steam. Lean over the bowl and inhale deeply. This provides instant relief to headaches, tiredness, stuffy nose and cold and flu symptoms.

Essential Oils for Headache

This is the best recipe to massage on the forehead area to relieve the pain instantly. It also helps with stress reduction and reduces headache.

Ingredients

1 tablespoon Peppermint essential oil

2 tablespoons Lavender essential oil

1 tablespoons Roman Chamomile essential oil

How to Use

Combine all the listed ingredients in a small bowl and then message on neck, shoulders and forehead for best results.

Oils for Body Aches

Ingredients

10 drops of lavender essential oil

2 tablespoons Roman Chamomile essential oil

2 tablespoons of Sweet Marjoram essential oil

How to Use

Mix all the ingredients and message the desire area. This recipe helps in soothing the aches and pains. It is also a great recipe to use before bedtime as chamomile will help you relax and sleep well.

The Massage Oil for Muscle Cramps

You can use combination of any of the below listed oil for cramps. Simply massage the area of concern for few minutes.

Oils

Essential Oils useful for cramps are:

Chamomile

Cypress

Basil

Carrot Seed

Lavender

Marjoram

Nutmeg

Peppermint

Rosemary

How to Use

All of the above mentioned oils have been known for relaxation qualities. So, you have complete freedom of choosing any of them or mix up any combination. The key lies in massaging the area correctly and not at an angle that will in turn cause more harm. After the massage is done, try to keep the muscle warm by wrapping a blanket etc. around you in order to assist the muscle in gaining the normal function again.

Skin Toner

4 oz. Green Tea (brewed) at room temperature

4 drops Lavender essential oil

6 drops Geranium essential oil

How to make and use

This recipe balances the pH level of the skin. The presence of antioxidants present in green tea has proven this recipe very effective. What you need to do is to combine the oils with the tea and shake them well. Then use the cotton pad to apply on face and neck. Repeat daily and see the difference.

Relaxing Bath

Another great mix to provide relaxation to whole body.

Ingredients

3 oz. of Honey

10 drops Lavender essential oil

How to use

Both of these ingredients can be directly added to a bath tub full of warm water. Honey is sure to soothe your skin while lavender will work to relax you during and after your hot bath.

You can also massage this blend all over your body before getting in the warm bath.

Thyme Oil for Relaxation

Ingredients

Thyme essential oil

How to use

Massage the oil all over your body and keep the body warm after the massage for at least 15 minutes to really experience the impact of the oil and the massage.

Conclusion

With this book in your hands, you can start dreaming about a beautiful you and actually work towards achieving the skin and hair of your dreams. This comprehensive book provides recipes for some simple, homemade easy to use skin, face, body and hair products. Therefore, fill up the void that has been created by the dissatisfaction caused by the commercial skin and hair care products. All the recipes are simple; contain organic and natural ingredients. These recipes are only basic combinations so don't be scared to experiment and create some of your own combinations. Natural is healthy and best for our body so don't be intimidated by the vast variety of options and ingredients you have at your disposal. Use this book as a guide and start the journey to a beautiful you.

Thank you for your purchase and being a part of this journey with me.

Like my page on facebook & get notifications for all of my upcoming ventures.

https://www.facebook.com/pages/Sarah-Reed/1401671063427858

Best Sellers by Sarah Reed:

Unleash the Power of Juicing
Lactose Free Smoothie Recipes